Multiple True/False Questions for the Primary FRCA:
Physics, Clinical Measurement and Data Interpretation

Simon A. May

CONTENTS

INTRODUCTION

At the time of writing, the MCQ component of the Primary FRCA examination comprises 90 multiple choice questions, to be completed within 3 hours. 30 of these questions are single best answer (SBA) questions and the remaining 60 questions are multiple true/false (MTF) questions. The MTF questions are designed to test theoretical knowledge, whereas the SBA questions will require you to apply this knowledge.

The 60 MTF questions are subdivided, approximately, as follows:
- 20 MTF questions in pharmacology
- 20 MTF questions in physiology and anatomy
- 20 MTF questions in physics, clinical measurement and data interpretation.

Each MTF question consists of a stem followed by 5 statements, each of which requires a true or false answer.

The questions in this book are based on the knowledge required for the MTF physics, data interpretation and clinical measurement component of the Primary FRCA MCQ exam. The SBA and other MTF components of the Primary FRCA MCQ exam are covered in separate books in the *Revise Anaesthesia* series.

The breadth and style of the questions mirror the Primary FRCA MCQ exam and for each question, there is a concise explanation. The questions are arranged into groups of 20 questions, followed by the answers and explanations for those questions.

MCQ books are an essential aid to FRCA exam revision. They quickly identify gaps in knowledge and therefore help focus future revision. The *Revise Anaesthesia* series differs from other MCQ books, as you are able to purchase questions separately for each component of the exam. This allows the books to be used as part of topic-specific revision and provides an alternative to expensive subscription-based question banks. Available in paperback and e-book format, the questions are yours to keep and access anywhere.

Best of luck in the examinations.

Questions 1-20

Q1:
The following are types of interval data:
A. Height
B. Age
C. Hair colour
D. Weight
E. Gender

Q2:
The following are colligative properties of a solute:solvent interaction:
A. Depression of freezing point
B. Lowering of the saturated vapour pressure
C. Elevation of the boiling point
D. Alteration in the specific heat capacity
E. Alteration in the latent heat of vaporisation

Q3:
The following units have the correct derivations:
A. 1 newton equals $1 \ kg.m.s^{-2}$
B. 1 joule equals $1 \ kg.m^2.s^{-2}$
C. 1 watt equals $1 \ kg.m^2.s^{-3}$
D. 1 hertz equals $1 \ s^{-1}$
E. 1 pascal equals $1 \ kg.m^{-1}$

Q4:
Regarding magnetic fields:
A. 1 tesla is equivalent to 1000 gauss
B. The Earth's magnetic field strength is approximately 5 tesla
C. Magnetic flux density is measured in webers
D. Moving a magnet through a coil of wires will induce an electromotive force
E. Fleming's left hand rule relates to the direction of force, magnetic flux density and current

Q5:
The following are appropriate tests for non-parametric data:
A. Mann-Whitney test
B. Wilcoxon Signed-Rank test
C. Kruskal-Wallis test
D. T-test
E. Analysis of Variance (ANOVA)

Q6:
Regarding common biological signals:
A. Electroencephalogram (EEG) has a frequency range of 0-100Hz
B. Electrocardiogram (ECG) has a voltage range of 0.1-50mV
C. Electromyogram (EMG) has a frequency range of 0-1000Hz
D. Electroencephalogram (EEG) has a voltage range of 1-500mV
E. Electrocardiogram (ECG) has a frequency range of 0-100Hz

Q7:
The following statements regarding capacitors and capacitance are correct:
A. Capacitors consist of two metal plates separated by a dielectric
B. Capacitance is measured in farads
C. One farad is equal to one coulomb per volt
D. The magnitude of charge on the plates is proportional to the voltage
E. Capacitors allow direct current to pass but block alternating current

Q8:
The following statements about the Clark electrode are correct:
A. It measures the partial pressure of oxygen
B. It contains a negative platinum cathode
C. It contains a positive silver/silver chloride anode
D. Potassium hydroxide is used as the electrolyte solution
E. It does not require a voltage to be applied

Q9:
The following pin index positions and medical gasses correctly match:
A. Oxygen and pin index numbers 1 and 5
B. Nitrous oxide and pin index numbers 3 and 5
C. Carbon dioxide and pin index numbers 2 and 5
D. Entonox and pin index number 7
E. Air and pin index numbers 1 and 4

Q10:

The following statements regarding oxygen are correct:

A. ISO and British standards store oxygen in a white cylinder with a black shoulder
B. A full oxygen cylinder has a cylinder pressure of 13700kPa
C. It has a critical temperature of 118°C
D. It has a boiling point of -183°C at 1 atmosphere
E. Gas separation occurs at -6°C

Q11:

Carbon dioxide can be detected by the following techniques:

A. Raman spectroscopy
B. Mass spectroscopy
C. Paramagnetism
D. Katharometry
E. Ultraviolet absorption

Q12:

Which of the following are correct regarding the oxygen failure alarm installed on anaesthetic machines:

A. It is mounted downstream of the rotameter block
B. It has an audible alarm of more than 60db at a distance of 1m
C. Power for the device is derived from the oxygen supply pressure
D. It is activated when the oxygen supply pressure is less than 100kPa
E. The Ritchie whistle is an example of an oxygen failure alarm

Q13:

The following should be checked before a new anaesthetic is administered:

A. Suction
B. Breathing system
C. Gas supply
D. Scavenging
E. Monitors

Q14:

Sterilisation of equipment can be undertaken with:

A. Autoclaving
B. 70% alcohol
C. Ethylene oxide
D. 2% gluteraldehyde
E. Gamma irradiation

Q15:

At 1 atmosphere the following statements are correct:

A. Water will freeze at 16 Fahrenheit
B. Water will freeze at 273.16 Kelvin
C. Water will boil at 212 Fahrenheit
D. Water will boil at 373.15 Kelvin
E. Water will boil at 100°C

Q16:

The following are approximately equivalent to 100kPa:

A. 1 atm
B. 10 bar
C. 2090 psi
D. 10400 dyne.cm^{-2}
E. 750 mmHg

Q17:

The following statements are correct concerning the Galvanic fuel cell:

A. Does not require a power supply to work
B. Has a gold mesh anode
C. Has a lead/lead oxide cathode
D. The electrolyte solution is potassium hydroxide
E. Lead reacts with hydroxyl molecules to form lead oxide, water and free electrons

Q18:

Which statements regarding thermocouples are correct:

A. They work on the principle of the Seebeck effect
B. The two metals most commonly used are copper and constantan
C. It has a relatively large output voltage change for increasing temperature
D. When the temperature difference between metals is $0°C$ there is no potential difference
E. As temperature increases the resistance reduces in a non-linear fashion

Q19:

Regarding laminar flow of a liquid in a tube:

A. The flow in the centre of the tube is twice the average velocity of the liquid
B. Flow is directly proportional to viscosity
C. Flow is directly proportional to increasing length
D. Flow is directly proportional to the diameter^4
E. Flow is directly proportional to the radius^2

Q20:

The storage of oxygen in a vacuum insulated evaporator (VIE) requires:

A. An inner temperature higher than the critical temperature of oxygen
B. An inner temperature below the boiling point of oxygen
C. A safety valve to prevent over pressurisation of the container
D. A pressure regulating valve for pipeline supply
E. A superheater to allow for "top up" supply

Q1:
A. T
B. F
C. F
D. T
E. F

Interval data is quantitative and continuous, i.e. height and weight.

Q2:
A. T
B. T
C. T
D. F
E. F

The colligative effects of a solution include a relative lowering in saturated vapour pressure, an elevation of boiling point and a reduction in freezing point.

Q3:
A. T
B. T
C. T
D. T
E. F

All the phenomena listed have the correct derived units except the pascal, which is force dissipated over 1 square metre (i.e. kgm^{-2}).

Q4:
A. F
B. F
C. T
D. T
E. T

Magnetic field strength is measured in teslas. 1 tesla is equivalent to 10000 gauss. The Earth's magnetic field strength is approximately 50 microteslas. Magnetic flux density is measured in webers and 1 weber is equal to 1 tesla per metre^2. Fleming's left hand rule relates to the direction of force, magnetic field and current for an electric motor.

Q5:
A. T
B. T
C. T
D. F
E. F

Tests for non-parametric data include: Chi-square test, Mann-Whitney test, Wilcoxon Signed-Rank test, Kruskal-Wallis test, Freidman's test and Spearman's test.

Q6:
A. F
B. T
C. T
D. F
E. T

Electrocardiograms (ECG) have a voltage range of 0.1-50mV and a frequency range of 0-100Hz.

Electroencephalograms (EEG) have a voltage of 1-500 mV and a frequency range of 0-60Hz.

Electromyograms (EMG) have a voltage of 0.01-100mV with a frequency range of 0-1000Hz.

Q7:
A. T
B. T
C. T
D. T
E. F

A capacitor consists of two metal plates separated by a dielectric. Capacitance is measured in farads with 1 farad being equal to 1 coulomb per volt. Charge is measured in coulombs and the charge a capacitor can contain is proportional to the voltage applied. Capacitors allow alternating current to pass but are relatively resistant to the flow of direct current.

Q8:
A. T
B. T
C. T
D. F
E. F

The Clark electrode measures the partial pressure of oxygen via redox reactions that occur at each electrode. It has a silver/silver chloride anode and platinum cathode and uses potassium chloride as the electrolyte solution. The galvanic cell utilises potassium hydroxide as the electrolyte solution and has a gold mesh cathode and lead/lead oxide anode. Unlike the galvanic fuel cell, it requires a voltage to be applied.

Q9:
A. F
B. T
C. F
D. T
E. F

The pin index system (PIS) is a safety tool that prevents the wrong medical gas cylinder being connected to the anaesthetic gas ports. Nitrous oxide's PIS is 3 and 5, oxygen's PIS is 2 and 5, air has the PIS of 1 and 5, carbon dioxide's PIS is 1 and 6 and entonox has the PIS of 7.

Q10:
A. F
B. T
C. F
D. T
E. F

Oxygen is stored according to British and ISO standards in black cylinders with white shoulders. When full, the cylinder pressure is 13700kPa (1980psi). As the cylinder only contains oxygen, there is no separation (unlike entonox cylinders). Oxygen has a critical temperature of -118°C and a boiling point of -183°C at 1 atmosphere.

Q11:
A. T
B. T
C. F
D. T
E. F

Carbon dioxide can be detected with Raman spectroscopy, mass spectroscopy and katharometry (thermal conductivity).

Q12:
A. F
B. T
C. T
D. F
E. T

The oxygen failure alarm is a mandatory piece of equipment that is built into anaesthetic machines. It is mounted upstream of the rotameters and when the oxygen supply pressure falls below 200kPa, it activates an alarm of more than 60db, which is audible at a distance of 1m. The Ritchie whistle is an example of an oxygen failure alarm.

Q13:
A. T
B. T
C. F
D. F
E. F

The Association of Anaesthetists of Great Britain and Ireland (AAGBI) have released a document detailing how anaesthetic equipment should be checked. At the start of every new session the power supply, gas supply, suction, breathing system, ventilator, scavenging, monitors and airway equipment should be checked. Between each new case the breathing system, ventilator, airway equipment and suction should be checked.

Q14:

A. T
B. F
C. T
D. F
E. T

Sterilisation requires the killing of all micro-organisms and can be undertaken with gamma irradiation, autoclaving, ethylene oxide and a dry heat. Disinfection (killing non spore-forming organisms) can be undertaken with 2% gluteraldehyde, 70% alcohol, hydrogen peroxide, phenol or pasteurisation.

Q15:

A. F
B. F
C. T
D. T
E. T

The freezing point of water occurs at 0°C, 32F or 273.15K at 1 atmosphere. The boiling point of water is 100°C, 212F or 373.15K at 1 atmosphere. The triple point of water occurs at 273.16K.

Q16:

A. T
B. F
C. F
D. T
E. T

100kPa is approximately equivalent to 1 atm, 1 bar, 750mmHg, 1020cmH$_2$O, 14.5psi or 10400dyne.cm^{-2}.

Q17:
A. T
B. F
C. F
D. T
E. T

The Galvanic fuel cell has a lead/lead oxide anode, a gold cathode and is in a potassium hydroxide electrolyte. It does not require a power supply and the detection of the current produced by the reaction is a marker of oxygen partial pressure.

At the lead anode: $2Pb + 4OH^- = PbO + H_2O + 2e^-$.

Q18:
A. T
B. T
C. F
D. T
E. F

The thermocouple works on the Seebeck principle, which states that two dissimilar metals produce a potential difference when they are at different temperatures. The thermocouple produces relatively small voltages for an increase in temperature and the common metals are copper and constantan. In a thermistor, the resistance falls in a linear fashion with increasing temperature.

Q19:
A. T
B. F
C. F
D. T
E. F

Laminar flow is governed by the Hagen-Poiseuille equation. Flow is directly proportional to the pressure difference, radius^4 or the diameter^4. It is inversely proportional to the viscosity and length of tubing.

Q20:
A. F
B. F
C. T
D. T
E. T

The vacuum insulated evaporator (VIE) stores oxygen below its critical temperature and above its boiling point at 1 atmosphere. This allows a mixture of liquid and gaseous oxygen (in equilibrium) to be formed, limits the pressure in the container and optimises the amount that can be stored. A safety valve is required and at times of peak demand a superheater is required to allow more gaseous oxygen to become available.

Q21:

Concerning the reaction of carbon dioxide and soda lime:

A. It is an endothermic process
B. Sodium hydroxide is a catalyst for the reaction
C. Water is a by product of the reaction
D. Calcium carbonate is formed from both soda lime and baralyme
E. Decreasing the surface area of the granules will improve carbon dioxide removal

Q22:

Concerning haemoglobin absorption spectra:

A. Has an isobestic point at a wavelength of approximately 800nm
B. Red light is better absorbed by oxygenated haemoglobin molecules
C. Absorption of light is indirectly proportional to the concentration of the medium
D. Absorption of light is indirectly proportional to the path length
E. Infra-red light has a wavelength greater than 850nm

Q23:

Saturated vapour pressure of a gas is increased by:

A. Increasing the temperature
B. Increasing the surface area of the liquid/air interface
C. Increasing the removal of molecules from the liquid/air interface
D. Oscillation of the surface
E. Bubbling a separate gas through the liquid

Q24:
Regarding vaporisers:
A. Anaesthetic vapour pressure equals the vapour pressure divided by the ambient pressure
B. Plenum vaporisers have a low internal resistance
C. Draw-over vaporisers can be driven by the patient's respiratory effort
D. Temperature compensation can be achieved with bimetallic strips
E. Temperature compensation can be achieved with aneroid bellows

Q25:
Regarding the desflurane vaporiser:
A. The vaporiser heats the desflurane to above its boiling point
B. It has a different design to plenum vaporisers due to the very low saturated vapour pressure of desflurane at room temperature
C. Desflurane vaporisers achieve a saturated vapour pressure of 194kPa
D. The fresh gas flow is entirely separate to the vaporisation chamber
E. The vaporiser dial has a stop mechanism at 8% concentration

Q26:
The following are types of ordinal data:
A. Pain score
B. Eye colour
C. ASA anaesthetic risk score
D. Height
E. Blood group

Q27:

Concerning force, work and power:

A. Power can be measured in watts
B. Work done is equal to the force applied multiplied by the distance moved
C. 1 watt is equivalent to 1 joule per second
D. The force being applied to an object is the same as its mass
E. Force can be measured in newtons

Q28:

The following statements are true concerning injecting with a syringe:

A. The pressure generated is directly proportional to the force applied
B. The pressure generated is directly proportional to the cross sectional area
C. To maintain the same pressure, a syringe with a larger cross-sectional area requires a larger force to be applied
D. Doubling the cross sectional area requires double the force to depress the plunger
E. Halving the cross sectional area requires four times the force to depress the plunger

Q29:

Regarding gasses, liquids and solids:

A. The freezing point of a substance is independent of pressure
B. The boiling point of a substance is independent of pressure
C. Critical temperature is the temperature below which a gas cannot be liquified regardless of the pressure applied
D. It is possible for a substance to exist as a gas, liquid and solid at the same pressure and temperature
E. Vapour and gas are identical terms

Q30:

Concerning humidity:

A. Absolute humidity is the mass of water in a given volume of air
B. Relative humidity is usually expressed as a percentage
C. As temperature increases, relative humidity increases
D. Relative humidity is equal to the saturated vapour pressure divided by the actual vapour pressure
E. At 37°C 100% relative humidity would require an absolute humidity of 17gm^{-3}

Q31:

Regarding diffusion:

A. The rate of diffusion of a gas is directly proportional to the square root of the molecular weight
B. The rate of diffusion is directly proportional to the surface area of the interface
C. The rate of diffusion is directly proportional to the thickness of the membrane
D. The rate of diffusion is directly proportional to the concentration gradient
E. The amount of gas dissolved in a liquid is directly proportional to the partial pressure exerted by the gas on the liquid/gas interface

Q32:

Blood:gas solubility co-efficient:

A. Requires equal volume phases of blood and gas
B. Requires the blood and gas to be in a closed system
C. Is defined at a standard temperature
D. Is defined at a standard pressure
E. Relates to the potency of anaesthetic gasses

Q33:

Regarding resistors in an electrical circuit:

A. The total resistance of a circuit to resistors in parallel is additive
B. Resistance is defined as the ability to resist direct current
C. Impedance links resistance and reactance
D. Resistance is measured in coulombs
E. The resistance of a circuit is proportional to the voltage applied

Q34:

Regarding entonox cylinders:

A. Entonox is supplied in cylinders at a pressure of 137kPa
B. It is a 50:50 mixture of air and nitrous oxide
C. At high temperatures the gasses can separate
D. Comprise a blue cylinder with a white shoulder
E. Have a pin index number of 7

Q35:

Regarding the efficiency of different types of humidifier:

A. Cold water bubble through is the least effective method of humidifying gasses
B. Heated water baths are more effective than ultrasonic nebulisers
C. Ultrasonic nebulisers can lead to an overdose of humidity
D. An anvil nebuliser utilising the Bernoulli principle is ineffective compared to a heat and moisture exchanger
E. The efficiency of humidification of an ultrasonic nebuliser is related to the frequency utilised

Q36:

Concerning the behaviour of gasses:

A. At standard temperature and pressure, 1 mole of a gas occupies 2.24 litres
B. When multiple gasses exist together the total pressure exerted is additive
C. Increasing temperature will increase the pressure of a gas
D. Decreasing the volume will increase the pressure of a gas
E. Avogadro's number relates to the number of particles of gas that are present if the number of moles of the gas is known

Q37:

Advantages of the heat and moisture exchanger (HME) include:

A. Its ability to achieve 60-70% relative humidity
B. Its ability to achieve temperatures of 29-34°C
C. It decreases circuit dead space
D. It decreases resistance to flow by up to $2cmH_2O$
E. A microbial filter can be included

Q38:

Regarding Regnault's hygrometer and the dew point:

A. Consists of a silver tube containing alcohol
B. Utilises the condensation of water on the outer tubing to determine the dew point
C. The dew point represents the point at which ambient air is fully saturated
D. Allows for the deduction of relative humidity based on the temperature at which the dew point occurred
E. Requires a wick to encase the tubing

Q39:

When converting a substance from a liquid to a vapour:

A. Heat must be applied to change the state of a substance even though the temperature remains constant

B. Specific latent heat of vaporisation is the energy required to convert 1kg of a substance from a liquid to a vapour

C. Specific latent heat of vaporisation is constant regardless of the temperature of the substance

D. Latent heat of vaporisation for nitrous oxide is $0Jkg^{-1}$ at $36.5°C$

E. Latent heat of vaporisation is the key mechanism behind the principle of the cryoprobe

Q40:

When comparing the mercury and alcohol thermometer:

A. Mercury is a cheaper substance than alcohol

B. Alcohol is clinically safer than mercury

C. Mercury is more suitable than alcohol for recording low temperatures

D. Changes in alcohol with temperature are less linear than with mercury

E. Mercury is more suitable than alcohol for recording high temperatures

Q21:

A. F
B. T
C. T
D. T
E. F

The balanced chemical reaction for soda lime and CO_2 is as follows:

Step 1: $CO_2 + H_2O > H_2CO_3$
Step 2: $2NaOH + H_2CO_3 > Na_2CO_3 + 2H_2O + heat$
Step 3: $Na_2CO_3 + Ca(OH)_2 > CaCO_3 + 2NaOH + heat$

During this reaction, sodium hydroxide acts as a catalyst with heat and water being produced. Baralyme utilises barium hydroxide as a catalyst but calcium carbonate is still produced at the end of the reaction. Increasing the surface area of the granules will improve carbon dioxide removal but will also increase the resistance of the circuit.

Q22:

A. T
B. F
C. F
D. F
E. T

The Beer-Lambert law states the absorption of light is directly proportional to the concentration of the medium and the path length. The isobestic point for haemoglobin absorption of both oxygenated and de-oxygentaed species is around 800nm. Infra-red wavelengths are greater than 850nm. Red light is better absorbed by de-oxygenated haemoglobin molecules.

Q23:
A. T
B. T
C. T
D. F
E. F

Saturated vapour pressure (SVP) is increased with increasing temperature, increasing surface area at the air/liquid interface and by increasing the removal of molecules at the air/liquid interface. Bubbling other gasses or oscillating the liquid will not affect the SVP.

Q24:
A. T
B. F
C. T
D. T
E. T

Gas concentration supplied by a vaporiser is equal to the vapour pressure divided by the ambient pressure. Gas concentration can be too high, so manufacturers incorporate a splitting flow valve to limit this phenomenon.

If the liquid is vaporised too quickly (i.e. high gas flows) the temperature reduces. To compensate, bimetallic strips and aneroid bellows can redirect the gas flow to maintain the saturated vapour pressure. Plenum vaporisers have a high internal resistance. Draw over vaporisers have a low resistance hence can be driven by the patient's respiratory effort.

Q25:
A. T
B. F
C. T
D. T
E. F

The high saturated vapour pressure and low boiling point of desflurane requires a specially designed vaporiser. This heats the gas to 39°C (17°C higher than desflurane's boiling point), creating a saturated vapour pressure of 194kPa which is then placed into the fresh gas flow without the gas travelling through the vaporiser.

Q26:
A. T
B. F
C. T
D. F
E. F

Ordinal data is a subset of categorical data and implies ranking, such as ASA status or pain scores.

Q27:
A. T
B. T
C. T
D. F
E. T

Power is the rate of energy consumption and is measured in watts. 1 watt is equivalent to 1 joule per second. Work done is the total amount of energy expended and is the product of the force applied and the distance moved. Force can be measured in newtons but is not equal to simply the mass but that which is applied to the mass.

Q28:
A. T
B. F
C. T
D. F
E. F

Pressure in a syringe is equal to the force applied divided by the cross sectional area of the plunger. Therefore, pressure is directly proportional to force but indirectly proportional to cross-sectional area. Doubling the cross-sectional area requires increasing the force 4 fold to maintain the same pressure. Halving the cross sectional area reduces the force required. Hence, why it is easier to inject with smaller syringes than larger ones.

Q29:
A. F
B. F
C. T
D. T
E. F

The boiling and freezing point of a substance is influenced by the ambient pressure. It is possible for a substance to exist as a gas, liquid and solid at the same temperature and pressure and this is called the thermo-dynamic triple point. For water, this occurs at 0.006 atmosphere and 0.01°C. The critical temperature is the point below which a gas cannot be liquified regardless of the pressure applied. A gas is a substance that is normally in gaseous form at room temperature whereas a vapour exists as a liquid at room temperature.

Q30:

A. T
B. T
C. F
D. F
E. F

Absolute humidity is the mass of water vapour contained in a set volume. As temperature increases, the relative humidity decreases in a non-linear fashion. At 37°C the air has 100% relative humidity when it contains 44gm^{-3} water. Relative humidity is the actual vapour pressure divided by the saturated vapour pressure and is usually expressed as a percentage.

Q31:

A. F
B. T
C. F
D. T
E. T

- Graham's law states that diffusion is indirectly proportional to the square root of the molecular weight.
- Fick's law of diffusion states that diffusion is directly proportional to concentration gradient and area, but indirectly proportional to the thickness of the membrane.
- Henry's law states that the amount of gas dissolved in a solution is directly proportional to the partial pressure exerted by the gas at the liquid/gas interface at equilibrium.

Q32:
A. T
B. T
C. T
D. T
E. F

The blood:gas solubility co-efficient is the ratio of a gas between equal amounts of blood and gas at equilibrium in a closed system for a pre-defined temperature and pressure. It dictates the speed of onset of anaesthetic gasses.

Q33:
A. F
B. T
C. T
D. F
E. T

- Resistors in series have an additive effect.
- Resistance is defined as a circuit's ability to resist direct current, whereas reactance is the ability to resist alternating current.
- Impedance links resistance and reactance.
- Resistance is measured in ohms.
- Ohms law links voltage, current and resistance with voltage being directly proportional to resistance.

Q34:
A. F
B. F
C. F
D. F
E. T

- Entonox is a 50:50 mixture of oxygen and nitrous oxide.
- A full cylinder contains 137 bar of gas and is blue with a blue and white checked shoulder.
- At low temperatures the gasses can separate, initially causing ineffective analgesia as only oxygen is administered. When the oxygen is consumed only nitrous oxide remains which could potentially mean delivering a hypoxic gas mixture.
- Entonox has a pin index number of 7.

Q35:
A. T
B. F
C. T
D. F
E. T

Cold water bubble through is the least effective method of humidifying gasses followed by the heat and moisture exchanger (HME), heated water bath, anvil nebuliser and finally the ultrasonic nebuliser. The amount of humidity supplied by an ultrasonic nebuliser is related to the frequency and overdosage of humidified gas is possible.

Q36:
A. F
B. T
C. T
D. T
E. T

Dalton's law states that the partial pressures exerted by individual gasses is additive. At standard temperature and pressure, 1 mole of a gas will occupy 22.4 litres of space. Increasing temperature increases the pressure, as does decreasing the volume. Avogadro's number is the number of molecules present in 1 mole.

Q37:
A. T
B. T
C. F
D. F
E. T

The heat and moisture exchanger (HME) achieves relative humidity of 60-70% and is able to heat gas to 29-34°C. It increases the resistance of the circuit and increases the dead space. A microbial filter is often also added to the HME.

Q38:
A. F
B. T
C. T
D. T
E. F

Regnault's hygrometer is a silver tube which contains ether and has air bubbled through it. This causes cooling, resulting in condensation forming on the outer tubing. The temperature this occurs at is the dew point and corresponds to 100% humidity at the temperature concerned. From this information, relative humidity can be calculated. This type of hygrometer does not require a wick.

Q39:
A. T
B. T
C. F
D. T
E. T

To change a substance from a liquid to a gas, energy needs to be added (which does not change the temperature), this is termed the latent heat of vaporisation. The amount of energy required to change a substance from a liquid to a gas reduces with increasing temperature. The critical temperature of nitrous oxide is 36.5°C therefore the latent heat required is zero because it cannot exist as a liquid. The cryoprobe works on the principle of converting a liquid to a gas. This consumes latent heat and therefore cools whatever it is directed at.

Q40:
A. F
B. T
C. F
D. T
E. T

Mercury thermometers are clinically more dangerous and more expensive than alcohol thermometers. However, they have a better linear relationship to increasing temperature than alcohol thermometers. Due to mercury freezing at -39°C, alcohol is better for measuring low temperatures. Likewise, alcohol boils at 78°C, so mercury is better for monitoring high temperatures.

Q41:

The following are examples of azeotropes:

A. Halothane and ether
B. Alcohol and water
C. Petrol and water
D. Lipid and water
E. Sevoflurane and nitrous oxide

Q42:

The following are types of nominal data:

A. Gender
B. Blood group
C. Height
D. Pain score
E. Eye colour

Q43:

Regarding the properties of nitrous oxide:

A. At 40°C, irrespective of the volume or pressure, nitrous oxide exists only as a gas
B. At 36.5°C nitrous oxide has a critical pressure of 73 bar
C. At 20°C and 52 bar an equilibrium exists between liquid and gaseous nitrous oxide
D. At 20°C, dependant on the volume and pressure, nitrous oxide could be a gas, liquid or vapour
E. At 40°C nitrous oxide complies with Boyle's law

Q44:

The following statements are true concerning the normal distribution and skewness (kurtosis):

A. The standard normal distribution has a kurtosis of zero
B. Positively skewed data has a mode which is less than the median
C. Positively skewed data has a mean which is higher than the median
D. The standard normal distribution is defined as having a mean equal to zero
E. A value 2 standard deviations above the mean is at the 97.5 centile

Q45:

Regarding the standard deviation of a normal distribution:

A. 68% of values are within 1 standard deviation of the mean
B. 95% of values are within 2 standard deviations of the mean
C. 99.7% of values are within 3 standard deviations of the mean
D. Standard deviation is denoted by the greek letter omega
E. The standard deviation is the same as the square root of the variance

Q46:

Regarding the standard deviation (SD) and variance of data:

A. SD can only be calculated if the mean of the data is known
B. The formula for the SD is the same for whole population data and sample population data
C. SD requires a calculation of the variance
D. Variance can be defined as the squared differences of the mean
E. Variance is denoted by the greek symbol kappa

Q47:

The following are examples of class II electrical equipment:

A. Electric kettle
B. Hairdryer
C. Garden power tools
D. Low voltage lighting
E. Washing machine

Q48:

Concerning oxygen cylinders:

A. D cylinders contain 170 litres of oxygen
B. J cylinders contain 6800 litres of oxygen
C. C cylinders have a nominal full weight of 2.5kg
D. CD cylinders have a pressure of 137 bar when full
E. CD cylinders have a water capacity of 4 litres

Q49:

Concerning heliox cylinders:

A. When full, they contain either 1780 or 8200 litres of heliox, dependant on cylinder size
B. Contain 79% oxygen and 21% helium
C. When full, have a cylinder pressure of 137 bar
D. Are brown cylinders with brown shoulders
E. Have a nominal outlet pressure of 4 bar

Q50:
Concerning nitrous oxide cylinders:
A. The pressure gauge accurately reflects cylinder content
B. Regardless of cylinder size, they are all pressurised to 44 bar when full
C. D cylinders contain 900 litres of nitrous oxide
D. The filling ratio of nitrous oxide cylinders varies between countries
E. Nitrous oxide is stored in both gaseous and liquid phase inside the cylinder

Q51:
The following are appropriate tests for parametric data:
A. Freidman's test
B. T-test
C. Analysis of Variance (ANOVA)
D. Pearson's test
E. Chi-square test

Q52:
Causes of over damping on an arterial line include:
A. Arterial spasm
B. Presence of air bubbles
C. Narrow tubing
D. Stiff non-compliant tubing
E. Presence of blood clots

Q53:
Regarding the stimulation of nerves:
A. The minimum current required to stimulate a nerve is termed the rheobase
B. The time required at twice the minimum current to stimulate the nerve is termed the chronaxy
C. Human nerve fibres share the same chronaxy
D. Coulomb's law states that the further the nerve stimulator is from the nerve, the higher the current that is required to stimulate the nerve
E. Less current is required when the nerve stimulator needle is acting as an anode rather than a cathode

Q54:
Regarding La Place's law:
A. The same equation applies to both cylinders and spheres
B. Wall tension is proportional to the radius
C. Wall tension is indirectly proportional to the pressure contained
D. The radius of the vessel is indirectly proportional to the pressure contained
E. Explains the phenomena of the pressure required to inflate a balloon

Q55:
Regarding the flow of a gas:
A. The Bernoulli principle only applies to gasses and liquids that are behaving in an ideal manner
B. Increasing the flow velocity increases the pressure
C. The Venturi effect utilises a constriction in a pipe to decrease pressure
D. The Venturi effect utilises a constriction in a pipe to decrease velocity
E. The anvil nebuliser utilises the Venturi effect

Q56:

A perfect gas should:

A. Completely obey Charles' law
B. Completely obey Boyle's law
C. Contain molecules of infinitely small size
D. Contain molecules that have no volume
E. Contain molecules which exert no attractive forces

Q57:

The universal gas equation:

A. Requires the universal gas constant (R) which equals $8.32 \, J \, ^{\circ}C^{-1}$
B. Can be used to assess the remaining amount of gas in an oxygen cylinder
C. Can be used to assess the remaining amount of gas in a nitrous oxide cylinder
D. Is derived from combining the three gas laws
E. Requires Avogadro's number which is $6.02 \times 10^{23} mol^{-1}$

Q58:

The following statements about the "number needed to treat" (NNT) are correct:

A. It is the average number of patients treated to prevent 1 bad outcome
B. The lower the NNT, the less effective the treatment
C. A negative value means that the drug causes harm
D. The NNT to reduce pain by at least 50% for 400mg of ibuprofen is 12
E. NNT has no units

Q59:

Regarding inductors:

A. They consist of a conducting wire wrapped around a ferromagnetic material
B. Inductance is measured in henries
C. They are used in defibrillators to smooth out current delivery
D. Inductors allow the passage of direct current but hinder the passage of alternating current
E. The current applied to an inductor induces a magnetic field

Q60:

Regarding defibrillators:

A. Contain a capacitor
B. Contain an inductor
C. Contain a step down transformer
D. Contain a rectifier
E. The stored energy is equal to ½ the capacitance multiplied by the voltage

Q41:
A. T
B. T
C. F
D. F
E. F

An azeotrope is a mixture that always vaporises in the same proportions as the volume concentrations of the components in solution. The classical examples are ether with halothane and water with alcohol.

Q42:
A. T
B. T
C. F
D. F
E. T

Nominal data is a subtype of categorical data and is data that has no mathematical hierarchy or relationship, i.e. gender, blood group and eye colour.

Q43:
A. T
B. T
C. T
D. T
E. T

Nitrous oxide can exist as a gas, liquid or vapour but its state is dependant on the interaction of pressure, volume and temperature. Complicating this is the critical temperature and pressure of the gas. Amalgamating all these principles you can draw an isotherm of nitrous oxide. All the details in the data correlate correctly to nitrous oxide's isotherm.

Q44:
A. T
B. T
C. T
D. T
E. T

The normal (Gaussian) distribution is a bell shaped curve (i.e. unimodal) with a mean of zero. When it is symmetrical it is not skewed and the mean, mode and median are equal. If the peak is to the left it is positively skewed (positive kurtosis), with the mode less than the median which is less than the mean. A value 2 standard deviations above the mean will lie on the 97.5 centile.

Q45:
A. T
B. T
C. T
D. F
E. T

The normal distribution (bell shaped curve) has 68% of values within 1 standard deviation (SD) of the mean, 95% within 2 SD of the mean and 99.7% within 3 SD of the mean. Standard deviation is denoted by the greek letter sigma (σ) and it can be defined as the square root of the variance.

Q46:
A. T
B. F
C. T
D. T
E. F

Standard deviation (SD) requires a knowledge of the mean and the variance. The equation for calculating the SD of data is slightly different between data where the whole population or part of the population is sampled. As variance is the square root of the SD, it is given the symbol of σ^2. Variance can be defined as the squared difference of the mean.

Q47:
A. F
B. T
C. T
D. F
E. F

- Kettles and washing machines are examples of class I equipment (they are earthed).
- Class II equipment is double insulated to prevent inadvertent electrocution (examples include hairdryers and garden power tools).
- Low voltage lighting is an example of class III equipment (supplied from a separated/safety extra-low voltage (SELV) power source). The voltage from a SELV supply is low enough that under normal conditions a person can safely come into contact with it without risk of electrical shock.

Q48:
A. F
B. T
C. T
D. F
E. F

- BOC oxygen specification states that a D cylinder contains 340 litres of oxygen and a J cylinder contains 6800 litres of oxygen.
- C cylinders have a nominal full weight of 2.5kg.
- CD cylinders have an integral valve and when full have a cylinder pressure of 230bar (unlike standard valve oxygen cylinders which are pressurised to 137bar) and contain 460 litres of oxygen. CD cylinders have a water capacity of 2 litres.

Q49:
A. T
B. F
C. F
D. F
E. T

Heliox consists of 79% helium and 21% oxygen. It comes in brown cylinders with a white and brown checked shoulder in either 1780 or 8200 litre capacities. The cylinders are pressurised to 200 bar and have an outlet pressure of 4 bar. Helium cylinders are entirely brown with a nominal content of 1200 litres and a pressure of 137 bar.

Q50:
A. F
B. T
C. T
D. T
E. T

Nitrous oxide cylinders, when full, are all pressurised to 44 bar and the filling ratio varies between countries because the ambient temperature of hotter countries could be the same as nitrous oxide's critical temperature. In the cylinder, the nitrous oxide is in equilibrium between the liquid and gaseous form, which means that the cylinder pressure does not reflect the changing contents of the cylinder. C cylinders contain 450 litres, D cylinders contain 900 litres and E cylinders contain 1800 litres. The largest available cylinder is a J at 18000 litres.

Q51:

A. F
B. T
C. T
D. T
E. F

Tests for parametric data include: T-test (paired and unpaired), Pearson's test and the analysis of variance (ANOVA) test.

Q52:

A. T
B. T
C. T
D. F
E. T

Arterial line traces can be over damped due to loose connections, air bubbles, kinks, blood clots, arterial spasm or the use of narrow tubing. Under damping occurs with stiff non-compliant tubing.

Q53:

A. T
B. T
C. F
D. T
E. F

Nerve stimulation requires less current if the needle is acting as a cathode rather than an anode. Nerve fibres come in myelinated and non-myelinated forms as well as in different diameters, therefore they have separate chronaxy. The definitions of coulombs law, rheobase and chronaxy are accurate in the statements.

Q54:
A. F
B. T
C. F
D. T
E. T

La Place's law for a cylinder:
wall tension = pressure inside cylinder x radius

La Place's law for a sphere:
wall tension = 0.5 x pressure inside sphere x radius

Therefore, wall tension is directly proportional to the pressure contained and the radius. The pressure contained is indirectly proportional to the radius.

La Place's law explains the change in pressure required to inflate a balloon.

Q55:
A. T
B. F
C. T
D. F
E. T

The Bernoulli principle states that increasing the flow of an ideal liquid will simultaneously reduce its pressure. This can be applied to the Venturi effect, where a liquid or gas comes to a constriction and the pressure drops, resulting in a higher flow rate. Anvil nebulisers utilise the Venturi effect.

Q56:
A. T
B. T
C. T
D. T
E. T

A perfect gas does not exist. However, if it where to exist it should obey all the gas laws perfectly. In addition, the molecules should be of infinitely small size, not have any volume and not interact with other molecules.

Q57:
A. T
B. T
C. F
D. T
E. F

- The universal gas law can be utilised to determine the contents of an oxygen cylinder (as all the contents are in the gaseous form), but not a nitrous oxide cylinder.
- It is an amalgamation of the three gas laws and the universal gas constant.
- It does not require Avogadro's number to complete the equation.

- The universal gas law states:

> pressure x volume =
> universal gas constant x number of moles x temperature

Q58:
A. T
B. F
C. T
D. F
E. T

- The number needed to treat (NNT) is a mathematical concept that states how many patients need to be treated in order for one of them to benefit compared to a control patient. The number needed to harm (NNH) is how many patients need to receive a treatment for one patient to be harmed. If the NNT is negative, then harm, not benefit is the outcome of the intervention.
- NNT has no units.
- The Oxford League Table of analgesic efficacy give 400mg ibuprofen a NNT of 2.4.

Q59:
A. T
B. T
C. T
D. F
E. T

An inductor consists of a ferromagnetic centre with a coil wrapped around it. When a current is applied to the wire it induces a magnetic field and hence a voltage, which opposes the rising current. Inductors allow the easy passage of direct current but oppose alternating current. They are used clinically to smooth out the electrical discharge of a defibrillator. Inductance is measured in henries.

Q60:
A. T
B. T
C. F
D. T
E. F

Defibrillator circuits contain a step up transformer, rectifiers, an inductor and a capacitor. The energy stored for defibrillation equals 1/2 x capacitance x voltage^2.

Q61:
Concerning resistance thermometers:
A. There is a non-linear relationship between temperature and resistance
B. Platinum is a suitable material for the thermometer
C. They cannot detect small temperature changes
D. They have a quick response time
E. Resistance decreases with increasing temperature

Q62:
Thermistors:
A. Can be manufactured from the oxides of manganese, zinc or cobalt
B. Increasing temperature reduces the resistance of the thermistor
C. Has a rapid response time
D. Does not require recalibration
E. Needs signal amplification for processing

Q63:
The following statements regarding the classification of electrical equipment are correct:
A. Type B equipment must have a leakage current of less than 10 microamps
B. Type BF and type CF equipment have a floating circuit
C. Type B equipment is suitable for direct connection to the heart
D. Type CF equipment includes ECG leads
E. Type CF equipment provides the lowest degree of protection from electrocution

Q64:

Regarding the design of electrical equipment:

A. Class I equipment requires an earth connection
B. Class I equipment must have a fuse which melts in the event of a fault
C. Class II equipment must have double insulation
D. Class III equipment has a maximum alternating current voltage of 60 volts
E. Class III equipment can be battery operated

Q65:

The following increase the risk of harm from electrocution:

A. High current
B. Cardiac current pathway
C. High current density
D. Use of alternating current
E. Short current duration

Q66:

Surgical diathermy:

A. Monopolar diathermy generates energy at up to 200kHz
B. Monopolar diathermy has a large area neutral electrode to increase the current density
C. Monopolar cutting requires a modulated waveform
D. Bipolar diathermy relies on a high current density between two points on forceps
E. Bipolar diathermy has a lower power output than monopolar diathermy

Q67:

Sound waves exhibit the following properties:

A. Audible sound waves travel through air at 3300ms^{-1}
B. They are longitudinal waves
C. Sound waves can be detected by the human ear at up to 200kHz
D. Ultrasound waves require a frequency greater than 1MHz
E. Sound wave speed is related to the Bulk modulus of the medium traversed

Q68:

Regarding the likelihood of developing laminar or turbulent flow:

A. Laminar flow is more likely with increasing viscosity
B. Laminar flow is more likely with decreasing density
C. Laminar flow is more likely with a Reynold's number of 20000
D. Turbulent flow is more likely with increasing diameter
E. Turbulent flow is more likely with increasing velocity

Q69:

The following are basic SI (Systeme Internationale) units:

A. Ampere
B. Mole
C. Newton
D. Second
E. Volt

Q70:

With regard to the Bland-Altman plot:

A. It is identical to the Tukey mean difference plot
B. It is identical to the Pearson's product moment correlation co-efficient
C. It can be used to assess the correlation between two investigations
D. It quantifies bias
E. It quantifies the range of agreement

Q71:

The Mapleson A circuit:

A. The corrugated hose should be approximately 110cm
B. It is the least efficient system for spontaneous ventilation
C. A fresh gas flow equal to alveolar minute ventilation prevents rebreathing
D. It can be used in infants and small children
E. The Lack modification enables exhaled gas to pass along the outer tubing

Q72:

The Mapleson C circuit:

A. Is identical to a Water's circuit
B. Can be used to resuscitate or transfer a patient
C. The fresh gas flow enters distal to the spill valve
D. Is available in a co-axial form
E. High fresh gas flows are required to prevent rebreathing in spontaneous respiration

Q73:

The Bain co-axial circuit:

A. Is inefficient during controlled ventilation
B. Is a co-axial version of the Mapleson A circuit
C. Fresh gas flow is delivered via the inner tubing
D. Requires a fresh gas flow rate of twice the minute volume during spontaneous ventilation to prevent re-breathing
E. The bag is attached to the outer tubing

Q74:

The Mapleson E circuit:

A. Is identical to an Ayre's T-piece
B. Has virtually no resistance during expiration
C. Demonstrates the adequacy of a patient's tidal volume during spontaneous ventilation
D. Can be modified with an open ended bag to form a Mapleson F circuit
E. Allows for easy scavenging of anaesthetic gas

Q75:

With regard to lasers:

A. All waves are in phase both in time and space
B. All waves travel in a parallel direction
C. All waves consist of the same wavelength
D. Category I lasers are the most dangerous
E. Shorter wavelength light is strongly absorbed causing heating to superficial tissue

Q76:

With regard to lasers:

A. Carbon dioxide lasers emit ultraviolet radiation
B. Neodymium-yttrium-aluminium-garnet (Nd-YAG) lasers emit infra-red radiation
C. Argon lasers emit blue-green light
D. Carbon dioxide lasers can be used for cutting and coagulation
E. Argon lasers can be used for repairing structures on the retina

Q77:
With regard to infra-red capnography:
A. Erroneous readings can occur if water vapour enters the side stream analyser
B. The optimum gas sampling rate for side stream analysis is 500mlmin^{-1}
C. There is the potential to cause burns with a main stream capnograph
D. Response time is faster with side stream analysis than main stream analysis
E. Molecules composed of two or more dissimilar atoms will absorb infra-red radiation

Q78:
The following gasses have a cylinder pressure of 13700kPa when full:
A. Air
B. Carbon dioxide
C. Entonox
D. Helium
E. Nitrous oxide

Q79:
With regard to paramagnetic analysers:
A. Diamagnetic molecules possess two unpaired electrons in their outer shell
B. The Pauling type of analyser contains a dumbbell containing nitrogen
C. They have a response time of between 1 and 5 seconds
D. Nitrous oxide can be detected by paramagnetic analysers
E. Paramagnetic molecules are attracted towards a magnetic field

Q80:
The Benedict-Roth spirometer:
A. Is relatively small and portable
B. Consists of a light bell that traps a volume of air over water
C. Can measure the functional expired volume in 1 second (FEV_1) of a subject
D. Can measure the functional residual capacity (FRC) of a subject
E. Can measure the vital capacity (VC) of a subject

Q61:

A. F
B. T
C. F
D. F
E. F

Resistance thermometers are made from platinum as it has a large temperature co-efficient and does not corrode. They are highly sensitive to temperature changes but have a slow response time. Increasing temperature causes an increase in resistance in a linear fashion.

Q62:

A. T
B. T
C. T
D. F
E. F

Thermistors are semiconductors manufactured from metal oxides including zinc, cobalt, manganese. They have a reducing resistance with increasing temperature and offer a fast response time. Thermistors need recalibrating but do not need signal amplification (this is required for thermocouples).

Q63:

A. F
B. T
C. F
D. T
E. F

- Type BF and type CF circuits are floating circuits.
- Type C circuits offer the highest protection form electrocution and have a maximum leakage current of 10 microamps.
- Type B equipment has a maximum leakage current of 100 microamps and is therefore unsuitable for equipment which connects to the heart.
- Examples of type CF equipment include ECG dots and pressure transducers.

Q64:

A. T
B. T
C. T
D. F
E. T

- Class I equipment requires a direct earth circuit, which in the event of a fault causes a fuse to melt.
- Class II equipment is double insulated to prevent accidental contact with a fault.
- Class III equipment relies on a low voltage which is either less than 60 volts for direct current or 25 volts for alternating current. Class III equipment can be powered by a battery or step down transformer.

Q65:

A. T
B. T
C. T
D. F
E. F

Electrocution is more harmful if the:
- current travels through the heart
- current is high
- current density is high
- current duration is long

Direct current (particularly at the frequency of 50 hertz) is more harmful than alternating current.

Q66:

A. F
B. F
C. F
D. T
E. T

Monopolar diathermy generates electricity at between 200kHz and 6MHz. The diathermy tip has a small area for high current density and travels to a large surface area neutral plate, which reduces the current density. Monopolar diathermy requires a sine waveform. Bipolar diathermy has a lower power output because the current travels between two points on a pair of forceps, which keeps the current density high.

Q67:
A. F
B. T
C. F
D. T
E. T

Sound waves are longitudinal and travel at 330 metres per second in air. The speed of sound is related to the density and the Bulk modulus of the medium. The human ear can detect frequencies between 2Hz and 20kHz. Medical ultrasound requires frequencies greater than 1MHz.

Q68:
A. T
B. T
C. F
D. T
E. T

Reynold's equation derives a dimensionless number which predicts whether flow is likely to be turbulent or laminar in nature. A number greater than 2000 is likely to be turbulent. According to Reynold's equation, increasing the diameter, velocity or density is likely to make flow turbulent. Increasing the viscosity is likely to make flow more laminar.

Q69:

A. T
B. T
C. F
D. T
E. F

There are seven basic units in the Systeme Internationale from which all other units can be derived. These are the second, metre, mole, ampere, candela, kilogram and kelvin.

Q70:

A. T
B. F
C. T
D. T
E. T

To assess if a new investigation is as good as the gold standard investigation then a Bland-Altman plot is the statistical test of choice. It is also known as the Tukey mean difference plot and allows for assessment of bias and range of agreement. Pearson product moment correlation co-efficient assesses how closely two variables are matched to a linear regression model and is denoted by the letter r.

Q71:
A. T
B. F
C. T
D. F
E. F

The Mapleson A circuit is the most effective circuit for spontaneous ventilation (requiring a fresh gas flow of alveolar minute ventilation if there are no leaks), but least effective for controlled ventilation. The Lack modification is a co-axial version of the Mapleson A which requires exhaled gas to pass along the inner tubing. This circuit's dead space is too high for use in infants and small children.

Q72:
A. F
B. T
C. T
D. F
E. T

The Mapleson C circuit is used to resuscitate and transfer patients as it is highly portable. It is relatively inefficient for both spontaneous and controlled ventilation, hence requiring a high fresh gas flow rate to prevent rebreathing. The fresh gas flow is distal to the spill valve and the bag is at the distal end of the circuit. There is no co-axial version of a Mapleson C circuit. A Water's circuit is a Mapleson C circuit with the addition of a soda lime canister.

Q73:
A. F
B. F
C. T
D. T
E. T

The Bain circuit is a co-axial version of the Mapleson D circuit. It is efficient for controlled ventilation but not spontaneous ventilation (where it requires twice the minute volume to prevent rebreathing). The inner tubing contains the fresh gas supply and the bag is attached to the outer tubing.

Q74:
A. T
B. T
C. F
D. T
E. F

The Mapleson E circuit is identical to an Ayre's T-piece and if a bag is added to the circuit it becomes a Mapleson F circuit (known as a Ree's modification). It has virtually no resistance to exhalation but you cannot assess the adequacy of a patient's tidal volume (as there is no bag to see moving). It is difficult to attach scavenging to this circuit.

Q75:
A. T
B. T
C. T
D. F
E. F

Lasers always emit monochromatic light, that is in parallel and has the same phase. Domestic lasers are graded between 1 and 4, with category 4 lasers being the most dangerous. Longer wavelength laser light is more avidly absorbed, which causes superficial heating.

Q76:
A. F
B. T
C. T
D. F
E. T

ND-YAG and carbon dioxide lasers emit infra-red radiation. Argon lasers emit a blue-green light. ND-YAG lasers are used for cutting and coagulation and argon lasers can be used for repairing the retina.

Q77:
A. T
B. F
C. T
D. F
E. T

Main stream analysers for carbon dioxide offer fast analysis but are bulkier than side stream analysers and have the potential to cause burns (they have an elevated temperature to prevent water vapour affecting the result). Side stream analysers have a water trap to prevent water interfering with the result as water will also absorb infra-red radiation. The side stream analyser has a gas flow rate of between 50-200mlmin^{-1}. Any molecule with dissimilar atoms will absorb infra-red radiation, carbon dioxide has strong absorption for light with a wavelength of 4.3mm.

Q78:
A. **T**
B. **F**
C. **T**
D. **T**
E. **F**

Oxygen, helium, air and entonox have cylinder pressures of 13700kPa when full. Carbon dioxide has a cylinder pressure of 5000kPa and nitrous oxide 4400kPa.

Q79:
A. **F**
B. **T**
C. **F**
D. **F**
E. **T**

Paramagnetic analysis utilises the principle that oxygen is attracted towards a magnetic field due to the fact that it has two unpaired electrons in its outer shell. These unpaired electrons can cause rotation of a freely suspended dumbbell containing nitrogen to ultimately detect the oxygen concentration (this is called a Pauling analyser). Nitrous oxide cannot be detected by this method. Paramagnetic analysers have a response time of 5-20 seconds.

Q80:
A. F
B. T
C. T
D. F
E. T

The Benedict-Roth spirometer is a large and non-portable device which is essentially a bell which entraps a known volume of air above a water trap. As the patient breathes, the bell moves up and down and this is recorded on a drum with a pen. From this device the FEV_1, vital capacity, inspiratory reserve volume and expiratory reserve volume can be detected. The functional residual capacity cannot be detected with this device.

Questions 81-100

Q81:
With regard to statistics:
A. The null hypothesis and alternate hypothesis are the same
B. Type I error requires a false acceptance of the null hypothesis
C. Type I error misses true differences
D. Type II error falsely rejects the null hypothesis
E. Type II error detects false difference

Q82:
The following prefixes are correctly matched:
A. Nano 10^{-9}
B. Micro 10^{-3}
C. Deci 10^{-1}
D. Kilo 10^3
E. Mega 10^9

Q83:
Regarding mass spectroscopy:
A. It separates ions based on their mass to charge ratio
B. Requires a high vacuum chamber
C. When bombarded by electrons, molecules can exist as different species
D. When bombarded by electrons, produces negatively charged ions
E. The heaviest ions are deflected the most

Q84:
The Oxford Miniature Vaporiser (OMV):
A. Is a draw-over vaporiser
B. Thermal buffering occurs with a glycol reservoir
C. Is made from stainless steel
D. Is not suitable for paediatric anaesthesia
E. Can be used in series to augment output

Q85:

The Epstein Macintosh Oxford (EMO) vaporiser:

A. Is designed for use with halothane and is damaged by ether
B. The vaporising chamber sits in a water bath which acts as a heat sink
C. Stripping and maintenance is complex
D. Weighs over 10kg when set up
E. In plenum mode is ideal for paediatric anaesthesia

Q86:

With regard to ultrasound:

A. Attenuation is the absorption of ultrasound energy by a tissue
B. A low acoustic impedance between two substances improves reflection
C. Scattered reflection occurs when ultrasound is reflected from an irregular surface
D. Specular reflection occurs when ultrasound reflects from a nerve block needle
E. Refraction of ultrasound occurs at the border of substances with a different acoustic impedance

Q87:

With regard to logarithms of the same base:

A. $\log(a) + \log(b) = \log(ab)$
B. $\log(1/a) = -\log(a)$
C. $\log(b/a) = \log(a) - \log(b)$
D. $\log(a^b) = a\log(b)$
E. $\log_{10}(1) = 1$

Q88:
Concerning the rotameter for gas flow measurement:
A. It has a fixed orifice
B. It has a fixed pressure across the bobbin
C. It requires calibration for different gasses
D. Electrostatic charge may alter the reading
E. A ball bobbin measurement is taken from the middle of the ball

Q89:
With regard to molecules in a gas:
A. Equal volumes of gas at the same temperature and pressure contain equal numbers of molecules
B. 1 mole of a gas contains 6.022×10^{23} molecules
C. 1 mole of a gas at standard temperature and pressure occupies 224 litres
D. 1 mole of nitrous oxide weighs 44g
E. The mole is defined as the number of particles in 0.12kg of carbon^{12}

Q90:
With regard to an exponential process:
A. After 3 half lives, 6.25% of the initial value is present
B. The time constant is the time taken to complete the decline, had the initial rate of change continued
C. The time taken for an exponential process to reach 0 is finite
D. The rate constant is the reciprocal of the time constant
E. The half life is equivalent to 0.693 of the time constant

Q91:

Regarding the time constant:

A. It is the reciprocal of the rate constant
B. It is the time taken for an exponential process to decline to 50% of its original value
C. It is the time taken for an exponential process to change by a factor of e^1
D. It is the time a negative exponential would take to complete, had the initial rate of change been maintained
E. 0.693 multiplied by the time constant equals the half life of the process

Q92:

The following are dimensionless numbers:

A. Density
B. Force
C. Length
D. Reynold's number
E. Viscosity

Q93:

The following can falsely alter the pulse oximetry value:

A. Atrial fibrillation
B. Excess ambient light
C. Hyperbilirubinaemia
D. Nail varnish
E. Skin complexion

Q94:

The pH electrode:

A. Is also known as the Severinghaus electrode
B. Relies on the potential difference generated by the hydrogen ion difference between the sample and control electrodes
C. The value obtained by the pH electrode is temperature dependant
D. The reading and reference electrodes are silver/silver chloride in nature
E. The reference electrode is separated from the blood by pH sensitive glass

Q95:

The following statements are correct regarding peripheral nerve stimulation to monitor neuromuscular blockade:

A. The electrical pulse generated should exceed 60mV to be supra-maximal
B. Tetanic stimulation requires a supra-maximal stimulus for 5 seconds at 50 Hertz
C. Double burst stimulation consists of two bursts of 50 Hertz stimuli separated by 500 milliseconds
D. Train of four monitoring is four stimuli over 2 seconds
E. A stimulus for train of four monitoring lasts 0.2 milliseconds

Q96:

The Doppler effect:

A. Describes how the frequency of sound is altered after being reflected from a moving object
B. The velocity of the object is directly proportional to the frequency shift
C. The velocity of the object is indirectly proportional to the sine of the angle of incidence
D. The velocity of the object is directly proportional to the speed of sound in the medium concerned
E. Requires knowledge of the initial emitted frequency

Q97:
British standards for an oxygen failure warning device include:

A. An alarm volume of greater than 40db, which is audible from a distance of 1m
B. An alarm that continues for 10s or more
C. Activation when the supply pressure falls below 200kPa
D. An alarm that cannot be reset until the oxygen supply pressure is restored
E. An alarm that maintains the anaesthetic gas supply to the patient in the event of oxygen failure

Q98:
The back bar of an anaesthetic machine:

A. Has a "blow off" valve which opens at 10kPa
B. Has a "blow off" valve to protect the patient from barotrauma
C. Has a normal outlet pressure of approximately 1kPa
D. Has a pressure at the rotameter end of approximately 10kPa
E. Pressure at the rotameter end is influenced by total gas flow

Q99:
The Von Recklinghausen oscillotonometer:

A. Measures both systolic and diastolic blood pressure
B. Requires the use of a stethoscope
C. Has two overlapping cuffs
D. The point of maximal needle amplitude correlates to the mean arterial pressure
E. Has a bleed valve and a control lever

Q100:
Regarding the maximum exposure to anaesthetic gasses:
A. It is derived as a time weighted average over 8 hours
B. Varies between the United Kingdom and United States of America
C. For nitrous oxide is 100 parts per million
D. For isoflurane is 5 parts per million
E. For halothane is 1 part per million

Q81:
A. F
B. F
C. F
D. F
E. F

The null hypothesis states that there is no difference between two groups, whereas, the alternate hypothesis states that there will be a difference between two groups. Type I error is the false rejection of the null hypothesis and therefore detects false difference. Type II error falsely accepts the null hypothesis, therefore causing true differences to be missed.

Q82:
A. T
B. F
C. T
D. T
E. F

Nano is 10^{-9}, milli 10^{-3}, micro 10^{-6}, centi 10^{-2}, deci 10^{-1}, kilo 10^3, mega 10^6 and giga 10^9.

Q83:
A. T
B. T
C. T
D. F
E. F

Mass spectrometers fire electrons at a molecule, causing it to split into charged molecules. Depending on the original molecule it can exist in many different positive charge and mass variants. These are then accelerated towards a plate in a vacuum and dependant on the mass and charge are deflected by varying amounts. When the compound hits the plate it can then be identified. Heavy molecules are deflected the least.

Q84:
A. T
B. T
C. T
D. F
E. T

The Oxford Miniature Vaporiser (OMV) is a highly portable draw-over vaporiser. It has a relatively small chamber (50mls) and is thermally buffered by glycol within a metal heat sink. The OMV is made from stainless steel and has metal wicks to increase the output (though this increases internal resistance). The OMV can be used in series with other vaporisers, as is the case in the tri-service military device. It is useful in paediatric anaesthesia.

Q85:
A. F
B. T
C. F
D. T
E. F

The Epstein Macintosh Oxford (EMO) vaporiser is designed for use with ether and is damaged by halothane. It is easily stripped and maintained with a weight of approximately 10kg when fully prepared. The heat sink is a water bath which can be emptied to improve transportability. In plenum mode, the vaporiser is only accurate with flows greater than 10lm^{-1} which makes paediatric anaesthesia non-ideal.

Q86:
A. T
B. F
C. T
D. T
E. T

Ultrasound waves are reflected back to the transducer at boundaries between materials of different acoustic impedance. The greater the distance, the less ultrasound is returned to the transducer. At the border of materials with a different acoustic impedance, refraction occurs. As ultrasound traverses a material its energy is slowly consumed and this is termed attenuation. Scattered reflection occurs on irregular surfaces and the ultrasound waves are dispersed in many directions leading to a poor quality image. When a straight edge reflects most of the waves back to the transducer (such as a nerve stimulator needle), this is termed specular reflection.

Q87:
A. T
B. T
C. F
D. F
E. F

Logarithms are a way of expressing large numbers. Logarithms have a base number (usually 10 or Euler's number), which is then to the power of whatever the variable is. Logarithms can only be combined if they share the same base. the following rules apply to logarithmic transformations:

- $\log(a) + \log(b) = \log(ab)$
- $\log(1/a) = -\log(a)$
- $\log(a/b) = \log(a) - \log(b)$
- $\log(a^b) = b\log(a)$
- $\log_{10}(1) = 0$
- $\log_{10}(10) = 1$
- $\ln(e) = 1$

Q88:
A. F
B. T
C. T
D. T
E. T

The rotameter has a variable orifice which maintains a fixed pressure across a bobbin when gas flow alters. Electrostatic charge can be created by the bobbin rubbing against the tubing which can alter the accuracy. Due to the different viscosities and densities of gasses, each rotameter needs special calibration for the gas concerned.

Q89:
A. T
B. T
C. F
D. T
E. F

The mole is defined as something with the same number of particles as is contained in 12g (0.012kg) carbon^{12}. Avogadro's hypothesis states that equal volumes of gasses at the same temperature and pressure contain equal numbers of particles and Avogadro's number is the number of particles present in one mole (which is 6.022×10^{23} molecules).
1 mole of nitrous oxide weighs 44g.

Q90:
A. F
B. T
C. F
D. T
E. T

- A half life is the time taken for the original value to decrease by 50%. After 1 half life the value remaining is 50% of the original, after 2 half lives the value is 25% of the original and after 3 half lives the value remaining is 12.5% of the original.
- The time constant is the reciprocal of the rate constant and can be defined as the time taken to complete the decline had the initial rate of change continued.
- 0.693 of the time constant is equal to the half life.

Q91:
A. T
B. F
C. T
D. T
E. T

The time constant has many definitions and relationships including:
- Being the reciprocal of the rate constant
- The time taken for an exponential process to decline to 37% of its original value
- The time taken for an exponential process to decline by a factor of e1
- The time taken for a negative exponential function to decline to 0 had the initial rate of decline been maintained
- Being related to the half life by a multiple of 0.693

Q92:
A. F
B. F
C. F
D. T
E. F

The only dimensionless number in this question is Reynold's number, which has no units assigned to it.

Q93:
A. T
B. T
C. F
D. T
E. F

Pulse oximetry values can be falsely altered by atrial fibrillation, arrhythmias, excess ambient light, infra-red contamination, low cardiac output states, nail varnish and different species of haemoglobin (methaemoglobin approximates the value to 85% and carboxymhaemoglobin to 90%). Severe anaemia can also change the value obtained.

Q94:
A. F
B. T
C. T
D. T
E. F

The Severinghaus electrode is a modified version of the pH electrode which is used to measure carbon dioxide.

The pH electrode comprises two silver/silver chloride electrodes, one of which is in a buffer solution surrounded by pH sensitive glass (reading electrode) and a reference electrode in potassium chloride solution. The relative hydrogen ion difference between the two electrodes generates a potential difference which is proportional to the pH difference. Importantly, this reaction is temperature sensitive.

Q95:
A. F
B. T
C. F
D. F
E. T

- The electrical pulse generated by a peripheral nerve stimulator to monitor neuromuscular blockade should be supra-maximal, which is usually defined as greater than 60 milliamps.
- Tetanic stimulation requires a supra maximal stimulus at 50 Hertz for 5 seconds.
- Double burst stimulation is two supra-maximal stimuli at 50 Hertz applied 750 milliseconds apart.
- Train of four monitoring is four stimuli over 1.5 seconds, with the first stimulus at t=0s, the second at t=0.5s, the third at t=1.0s and the final stimulus at 1.5s. Each stimulus for train of four monitoring lasts 0.2 milliseconds.

Q96:
A. T
B. T
C. F
D. T
E. T

The Doppler effect describes how the frequency of sound is altered after being reflected from a moving object and is utilised to determine the velocity of an object. The doppler equation states:

$$V = \Delta F \times C / 2 F_0 \cos\theta$$

V = Velocity of the object
C = Speed of sound in the medium concerned

F_0 = Frequency of the initial emitted sound wave

ΔF = Frequency shift, or difference in the emitted and received sound wave frequency

Therefore, velocity is directly proportional to frequency shift and the speed of sound in the medium concerned, and inversely proportional to the initial frequency and cosine of the angle of incidence.

Q97:
A. F
B. F
C. T
D. T
E. F

British standard BS4272 requires oxygen failure alarms to:
- Have an audible alarm of greater than 60 decibels at a distance of 1 metre for 7 seconds or longer.
- Activate when the supply pressure falls below 200 kilopascals
- Have power derived from the oxygen failure
- Be unable to be reset until the oxygen supply pressure is restored
- When activated, cuts off the supply of anaesthetic gas and opens the machine pipeline to air

Q98:

A. F
B. F
C. T
D. T
E. T

The back bar has a pressure of approximately 1kPa at the outlet end and 7-10kPa at the rotameter end. The rotameter end pressure is influenced by total gas flow, the vaporisers being used and the connections at the common gas outlet. A "blow off" valve exists to protect the machine (not the patient) and is triggered when the pressure exceeds 30kPa.

Q99:

A. T
B. F
C. T
D. T
E. T

The Von Recklinghausen oscillotonometer measures systolic, diastolic and mean arterial pressure without the need for a stethoscope. It comprises two cuffs, a large dial, a bleed valve and a lever to switch between the cuffs. The smaller cuff is used to amplify the pulsation of the artery and the larger cuff measures the pressure. The systolic pressure is the point where the needle on the dial starts to jump, optimal needle oscillation occurs at the mean arterial pressure and suddenly deteriorates as you approach the diastolic pressure.

Q100:
A. T
B. T
C. T
D. F
E. F

Removal of anaesthetic gasses and reducing the exposure to health workers is governed by the Control of Substances Hazardous to Health (COSHH) act. Excess exposure to anaesthetic gasses has been linked to spontaneous abortion (in females), male anaesthetists fathering daughters, decreased fertility and potentially liver, renal and haematological effects. The UK and USA have different values of maximum exposure but both are derived as time weighted averages over 8 hours. For halothane it is 10 parts per million, nitrous oxide 100 parts per million and isoflurane 50 parts per million.

Printed in Great Britain
by Amazon